Table of Cont

MW01268339

Muscles of The Face

Muscles of The Posterior Neck, Shoulders, and Thorax

Muscles of The Anterior Neck, Shoulders, Chest and Thorax

Muscles (Posterior View)

Muscles (Anterior View)

Front Muscles

Back Muscles

Muscles of The Shoulder & Back

Muscles of The Shoulder & Chest

Muscles of The Posterior Forearm

Muscles of The Anterior Forearm

Muscles of The Anterior Arm and Forearm

Muscles of The Posterior Arm and Forearm

Muscles of The Upper Limb

Muscles of The Lower Limb

Muscles of The Anterior Hip & Thigh

Muscles of The Posterior Hip & Thigh

Major Muscle From The Front

Major Muscle From The Back

Muscles of The Lower Leg

Muscles of The Leg (Calf) and Foot

Muscles of The Anterior Thigh

Muscles of The Posterior Thigh

Muscles of Abdomen

Neck and Shoulder Muscles

Name of Muscles

Neck and Torso Muscles

Muscles of The Neck

Muscle Types

Joints

And Many More....

Muscles of The Face

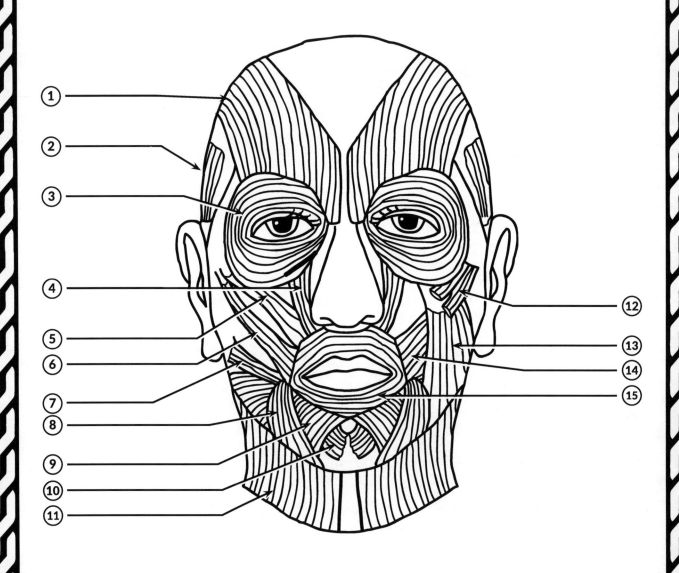

Muscles of The Face
- Answer -

(1). Frontalis

(2). Temporalis

(3). Orbicularis oculi

(4). Levator labii superioris

(5). Zygomaticus minor

(6). Zygomaticus major

(7). Risorius

(8). Depressor anguli oris (also called Triangularis)

(9). Depressor labii inferioris

(10). Mentalis

(11). Platysma

(12). Zygomaticus (cut)

(13). Masseter

(14). Buccinator

(15). Orbicularis oris

Muscles of The Posterior Neck, Shoulders, and Thorax

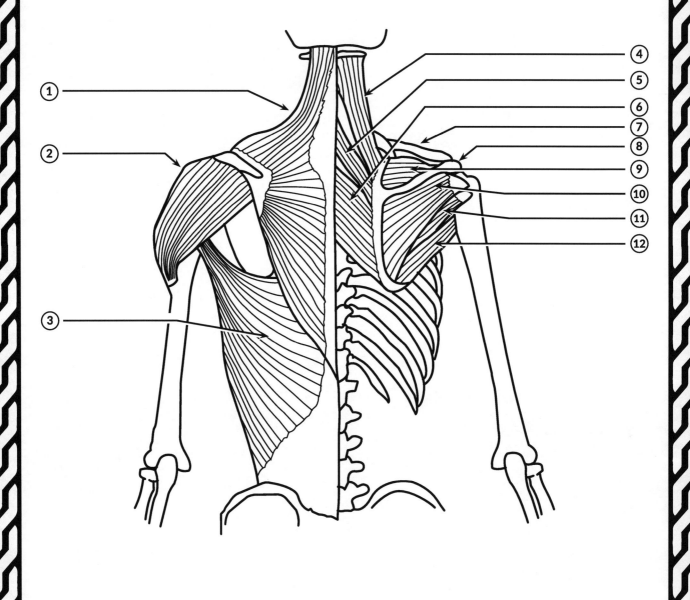

Muscles of The Posterior Neck, Shoulders, and Thorax

- Answer -

(1). Platysma

(2). Deltoid

(3). Latissimus dorsi

(4). Levator scapulae

(5). Rhomboid minor

(6). Rhomboid major

(7). Clavicle

(8). Scapular spine

(9). Supraspinatus

(10). Infraspinatus

(11). Teres minor

(12). Teres major

Muscles of the Anterior Neck, Shoulders, Chest and Thorax

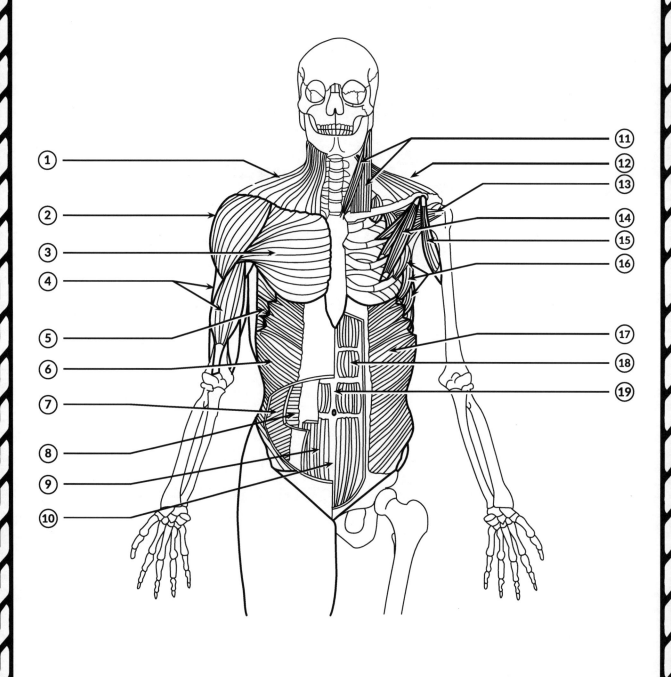

Muscles of the Anterior Neck, Shoulders, Chest and Thorax

- Answer -

(1). Platysma

(2). Deltoid

(3). Pectoralis major

(4). Biceps brachii

(5). Serratus anterior

(6). External oblique

(7). Internal oblique

(8). Transversus abdominus

(9). Rectus abdominus

(10). Linea alba

(11). Sternocleidomastoid

(12). Trapezius

(13). Subscapularis

(14). Pectoralis minor

(15). Coracobrachialis

(16). Serratus anterior

(17). External oblique

(18). Rectus abdominus

(19). Linea alba

Muscles
Posterior View

Muscles
Posterior View
- Answer -

(1). Flexor carpi ulnaris

(2). Extensor carpi ulnaris

(3). Extensor digitorum
Flexor retinaculum

(4). Gluteus medium

(5). Glutues maximus

(6). Adductor magnus

(7). Iliotibial tract

(8). Sartorius

(9). Semimembranosus

(10). Semitendinosus

(11). Biceps femoris

(12). Hamstrings

(13). Gastrocnemius

(14). Soleus

(15). Peroneus longus

(16). Achillestendon (Calcaneal tendon)

(17). Occipitalis

(18). Sternocleidomastoid

(19). Trapezius

(20). Deltoid

(21). Infraspinatus

(22). Teres major

(23). Rhomboid major

(24). Triceps brachii

(25). Latissimus dorsi

(26). Extensor carpi radialis longus

(27). Bracioradialis

(28). Flexor retinaculum

Muscles
Anterior View

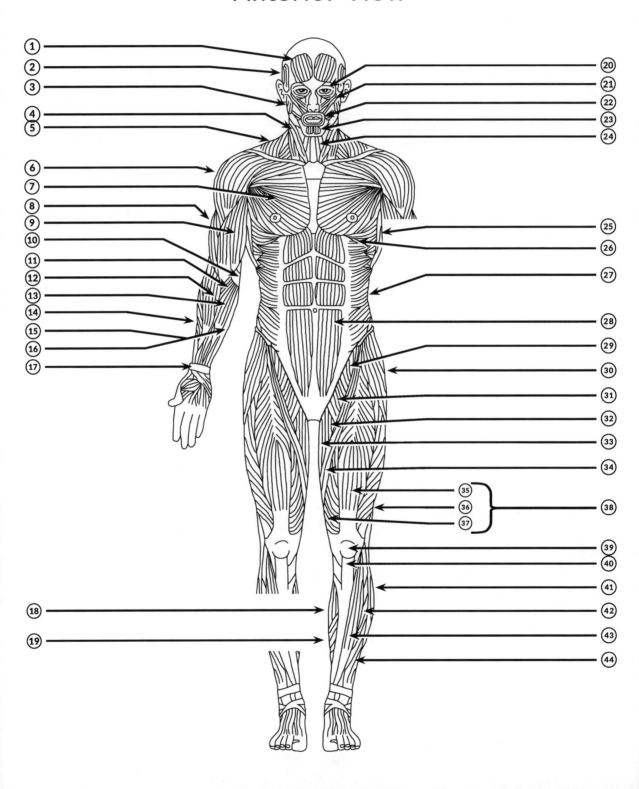

Muscles
Anterior View
- Answer -

(1). Frontalis

(2). Temporalis

(3). Masseter

(4). Sternocleidomastoid

(5). Trapezius

(6). Deltoid

(7). Pectoralis major

(8). Triceps brachii

(9). Biceps brachii

(10). Brachialis

(11). Pronator teres

(12). Brachioradialis

(13). Flexor carpi radialis

(14). Extensor carpi radialis longus

(15). Palmaris longus

(16). Flexor carpi ulnaris

(17). Flexor retinaculum

(18). Gastrocnemius

(19). Soleus

(20). Orbicularis oculi

(21). Zygomaticus

(22). Orbicularis oris

(23). Mentalis

(24). Sternohyoid

(25). Latissimus dorsi

(26). Serratus anterior

(27). External obliques

(28). Rectus abdominus

(29). Pectinius

(30). Tensor fasciae latae

(31). Adductor longus

(32). Adductor magnus

(33). Gracilis

(34). Sartorius

(35). Rectus femoris

(36). Vastus lateralis

(37). Vastus medialis

(38). Quadratus femoris

(39). Patella

(40). Patellar ligament

(41). Peroneus longus

(42). Extensor digitorum longus

(43). Tibialis anterior

(44). Peroneous tertius

Front Muscles

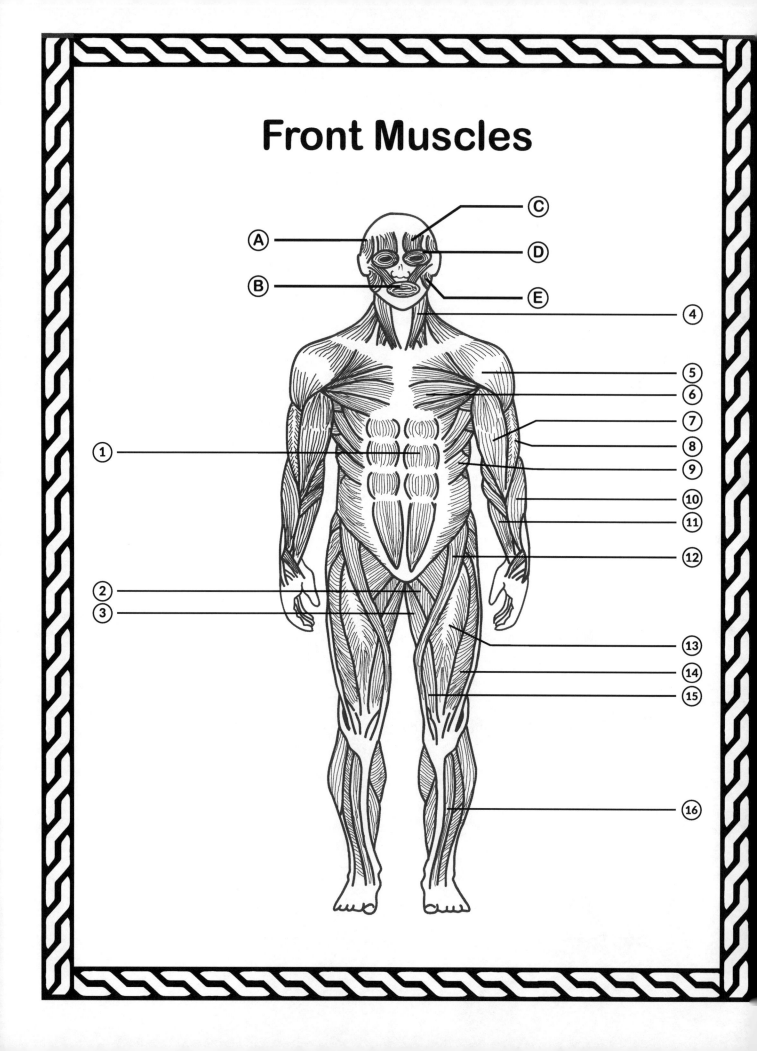

Front Muscles
- Answer -

(A) Temporalis

(B) Orbicular oris

(C) Frontalis

(D) Orbicularis oculi

(E) Masseter

(1). Rectus abdominis

(2). Adductor longus

(3). Gracialis

(4). Sternocleidomastoid

(5). Deltoid

(6). Pectoralis major

(7). Biceps brachii

(8). Brachialis

(9). External oblique

(10). Brachioradialis

(11). Finger flexors

(12). Sartorius

(13). Rectus femoris

(14). Vastus lateralis

(15). Vastus medialis

(16). Tibialis anterior

Back Muscles

Back Muscles
- Answer -

(1). Soleus

(2). Trapezius

(3). Infraspinatus

(4). Teres major

(5). Teres minor

(6). Triceps brachii

(7). Latissimus dorsi

(8). Finger extensors

(9). Gluteus medias

(10). Gluteus maximus

(11). Semitendinosus

(12). Biceps femoris

(13). Semimembranosus

Muscles of The Shoulder & Back

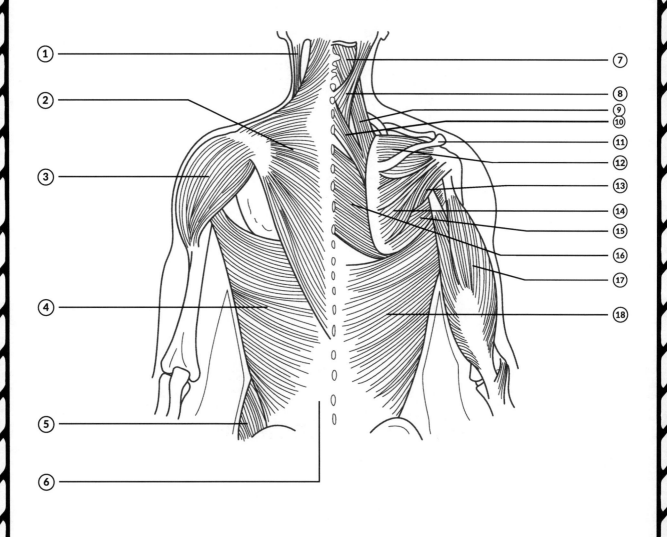

Muscles of The Shoulder & Back
- Answer -

(1). Sternocleidomastoid

(2). Trapezius

(3). Deltoid

(4). Latissimus dorsi

(5). External abdominal oblique

(6). Thoracolumbar fascia

(7). Semispinalis capitis

(8). Splenius capitis

(9). Levator scapulae

(10). Rhomboideous minor

(11). Acromion

(12). Supraspinatus

(13). Teres minor

(14). Infraspinatus

(15). Teres major

(16). Rhomboideous major

(17). Triceps brachii

(18). Latissimus dorsi

Muscles of The Shoulder & Chest

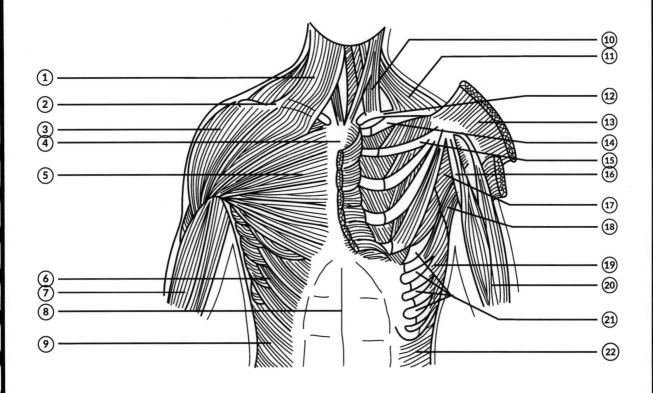

Muscles of The Shoulder & Chest
- Answer -

(1). Platysma

(2). Clavicle

(3). Deltoid

(4). Sternum

(5). Pectoralis major

(6). Serratus anterior

(7). Biceps brachii

(8). Rectus sheath

(9). External abdominal oblique

(10). Sternocleidomastoid

(11). Trapezius

(12). Clavicle

(13). Deltoid

(14). Subclavius

(15). Pectoralis minor

(16). Coracobrachialis

(17). Subscapularis

(18). Teres major

(19). Serratus anterior

(20). Biceps brachii

(21). Intercostal

(22). External abdominal oblique

Muscles of The Posterior Forearm

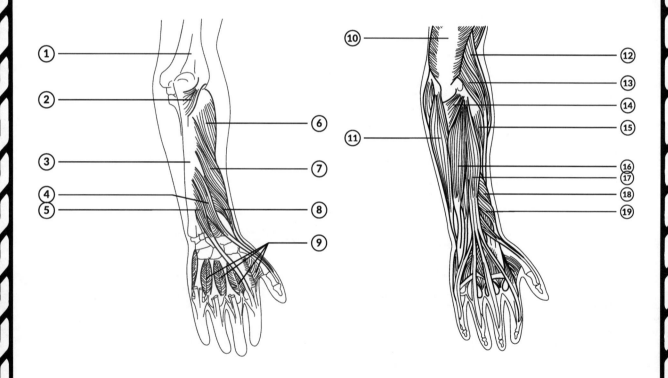

Muscles of The Posterior Forearm
- Answer -

(1). Humerus

(2). Anconeus

(3). Ulna

(4). Extensor pollicis longus

(5). Extensor indicis

(6). Supinator

(7). Abductor pollicis longus

(8). Extensor pollicis brevis

(9). Interossei

(10). Triceps brachii

(11). Flexor carpi ulnaris

(12). Brachioradialis

(13). Extensor carpi radialis longus

(14). Anconeus

(15). Extensor carpi radialis brevis

(16). Extensor carpi ulnaris

(17). Extensor digitorum

(18). Abductor pollicis longus

(19). Extensor pollicis brevis

Muscles of The Anterior Forearm

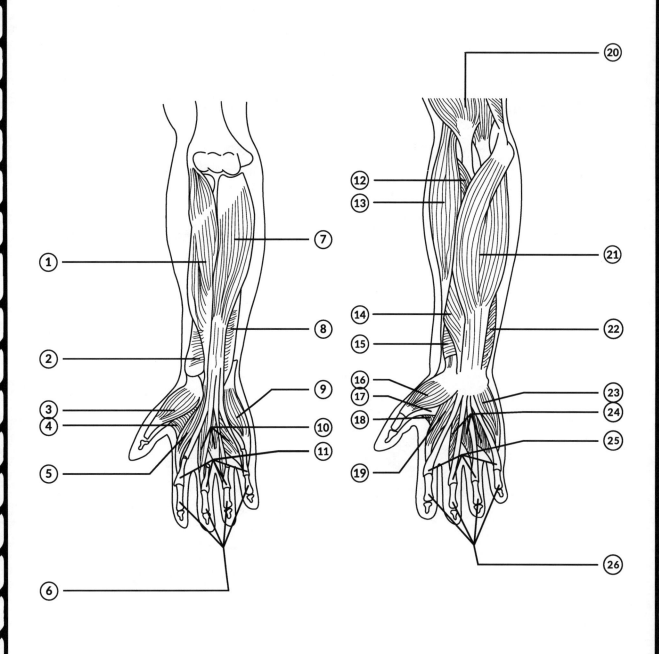

Muscles of The Anterior Forearm
- Answer -

(1). Flexor pollicis longus

(2). Pronator quadratus

(3). Thenar muscles of thumb

(4). Thenar muscles of thumb

(5). Lumbricals

(6). Flexor digitorum superficialis tendons

(7). Flexor digitorum profundus

(8). Pronator quadratus

(9). Opponens digiti minimi

(10). Lumbricals

(11). Flexor digitorum profundus tendons

(12). Supinator

(13). Extensor carpi radialis longus

(14). Flexor pollicis longus

(15). Pronator quadratus

(16). Thenar muscles of thumb

(17). Flexor pollicis longus tendon

(18). Thenar muscles of thumb

(19). Lumbricals

(20). Biceps brachii

(21). Flexor digitorum superficialis

(22). Pronator quadratus

(23). Opponens digiti minimi

(24). Lumbricals

(25). Flexor digitorum profundus tendons

(26). Flexor digitorum superficialis tendons

Muscles of Anterior Forearm

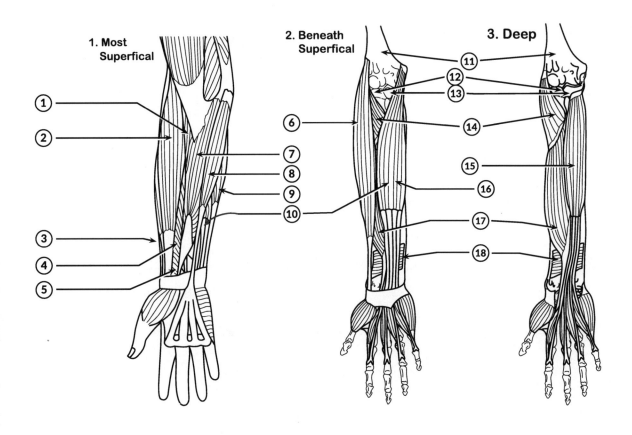

1. Most Superfical

2. Beneath Superfical

3. Deep

Muscles of Anterior Forearm
- Answer -

(1). Pronator teres

(2). Brachioradialis

(3). Extensor carpi radialis longus
(just visible here)

(4). Flexor pollicis longus

(5). Pronator quadtratus

(6). Extensor carpi radialis longus

(7). Flexor carpi radialis

(8). Palmaris longus

(9). Flexor carpi ulnaris

(10). Flexor Digitorum Superficialis
(deep to the above three muscles)

(11). Humerus

(12). Radius

(13). Ulna

(14). Supinator

(15). Flexor digitorum profundus

(16). Flexor digitorum superficialis

(17). Flexor pollicus longus

(18). Pronator quadratus

Muscles of the Anterior Arm and Forearm
(Most Superfical)

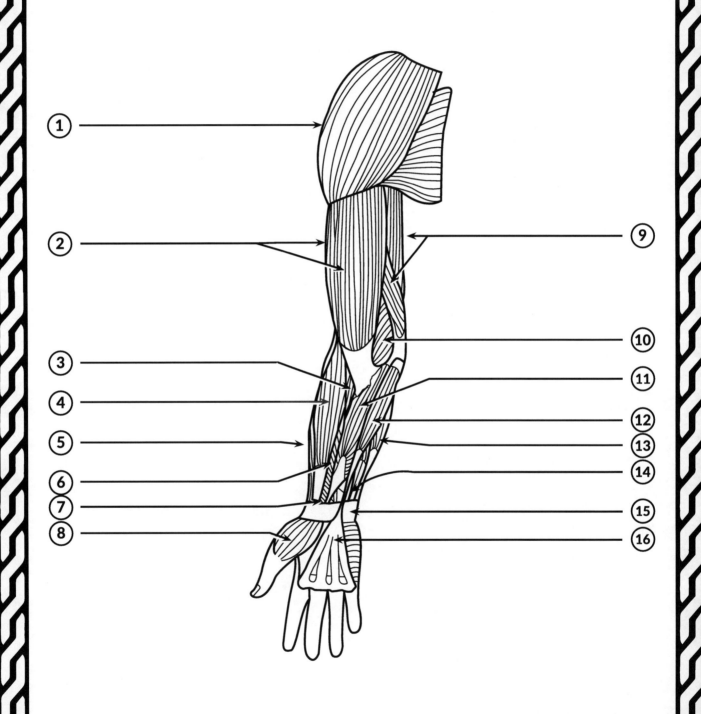

Muscles of the Anterior Arm and Forearm
(Most Superfical)
- Answer -

(1). Deltoid

(2). Biceps brachii

(3). Pronator teres

(4). Brachioradialis

(5). Extensor carpi radialis longus
(posterior - just visible here)

(6). Flexor pollicis longus

(7). Pronator quadratus

(8). Thenar muscles of the thumb

(9). Triceps brachii

(10). Brachialis

(11). Flexor carpi radialis

(12). Palmaris longus

(13). Flexor carpi ulnaris

(14). Flexor Digitorum superficialis
(deep to the above 3 muscles)

(15). Flexor retinaculum

(16). Palmar aponeurosis (fascia)

Muscles of the Posterior Arm and Forearm

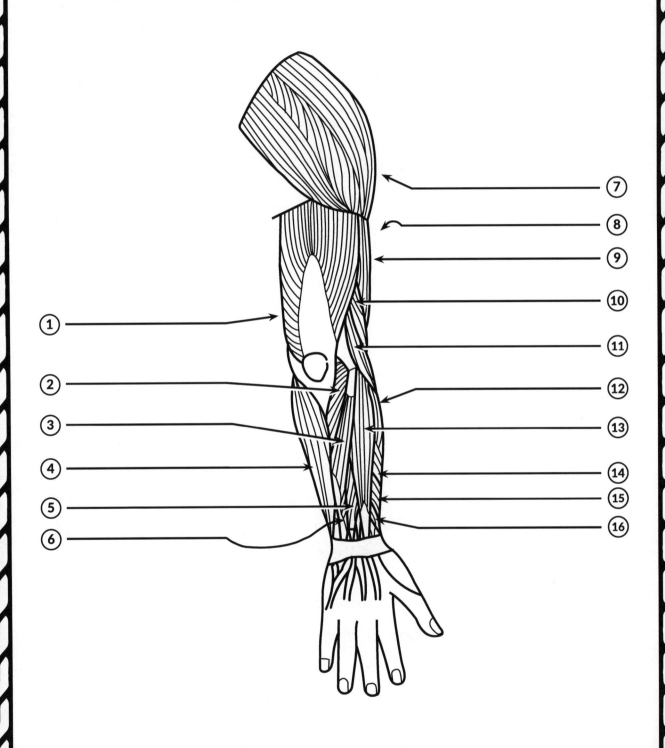

Muscles of the Posterior Arm and Forearm
- Answer -

(1). Triceps brachii

(2). Anconeus

(3). Extensor carpi ulnaris

(4). Flexor carpi ulnaris

(5). Extensor digiti minimi

(6). Extensor indicis (deep)

(7). Deltoid

(8). Biceps brachii (anterior)

(9). Brachialis

(10). Brachioradialis

(11). Extensor carpi radialis longus

(12). Extensor carpi radialis brevis

(13). Extensor digitorum

(14). Abductor pollicis longus

(15). Extensor pollicis brevis

(16). Extensor pollicis longus

The Muscles of The Upper Limb

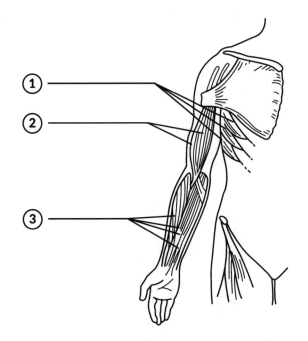

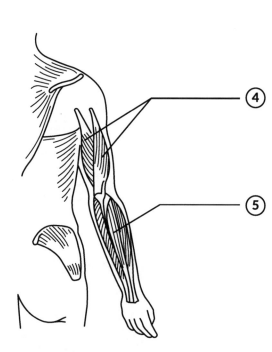

① ② ③ ④ ⑤

Anterior   **Posterior**

The Muscles of The Upper Limb
- Answer -

(1). Serratus anterior

(2). Biceps

(3). Wrist flexor muscles

(4). Triceps

(5). Wrist extensor muscles

The Muscles of The Lower Limb

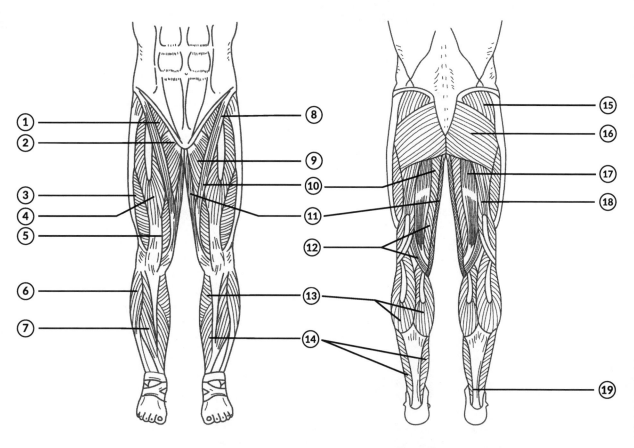

Anterior

Posterior

The Muscles of The Lower Limb
- Answer -

(1). Iliacus

(2). Pectineus

(3). Vastus lateralis

(4). Rectus femoris

(5). Vastus medialis

(6). Fibularis longus

(7). Tibialis anterior

(8). Sartorius

(9). Adductor longus

(10). Adductor magnus

(11). Gracilis

(12). Semimembranosus

(13). Gastrocnemius

(14). Soleus

(15). Gluteus medius

(16). Gluteus maximus

(17). Semitendinosus

(18). Biceps femoris

(19). Achilles tendon

Muscles of The Anterior Hip & Thigh

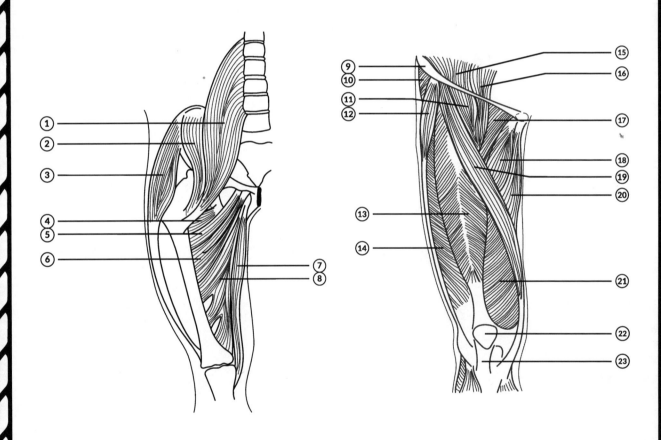

Muscles of The Anterior Hip & Thigh
- Answer -

(1). Psoas major

(2). Iliacus

(3). Tensor fasciae latae

(4). Adductor magnus

(5). Adductor brevis

(6). Adductor longus

(7). Gracilis

(8). Adductor magnus

(9). Inguinal ligament

(10). Gluteus medius

(11). Iliopsoas

(12). Tensor fasciae latae

(13). Rectus femoris

(14). Vastus lateralis

(15). Iliacus

(16). Psoas major

(17). Pectineus

(18). Adductor longus

(19). Sartorius

(20). Gracilis

(21). Vastus medialis

(22). Patella bone

(23). Patellar ligament

Muscles of The Posterior Hip & Thigh

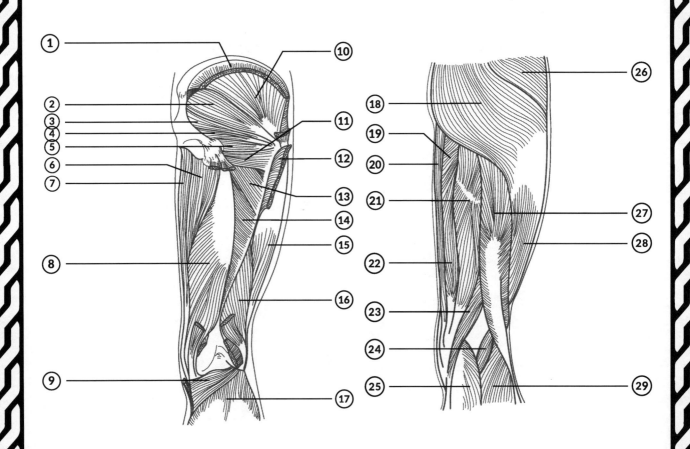

Muscles of The Posterior Hip & Thigh
- Answer -

(1). Gluteus medius

(2). Piriformis

(3). Superior gemellus

(4). Obturator internus

(5). Inferior gemellus

(6). Adductor magnus

(7). Inferior gemellus

(8). Semimembranosus

(9). Popliteus

(10). Gluteus minimus

(11). Quadratus femoris

(12). Gluteus maximus

(13). Adductor minimus

(14). Adductor magnus

(15). Vastus lateralis

(16). Biceps femoris

(17). Gastrocnemius

(18). Gluteus maximus

(19). Adductor magnus

(20). Gracilis

(21). Semitendinosus

(22). Semimembranosus

(23). Semimembranosus

(24). Plantaris

(25). Gastrocnemius

(26). Gluteus medius

(27). Biceps femoris

(28). Vastus lateralis

(29). Gastrocnemius

Major Muscle From The Front

1
2
3
4
5
6
7
8
9
10
11

Quadriceps femoris group

12
13
14
15
16
17

18
19
20

Adductor group

21
22
23

24
25

Major Muscle From The Front
- Answer -

(1). Frontalis

(2). Orbicularis oculi

(3). Zygomaticus

(4). Masseter

(5). Sternocleidomastoid

(6). Trapezius

(7). Deltoid

(8). Rectus abdominis

(9). External oblique

(10). Iliopsoas

(11). Sartorious

(12). Vastus lateralis

(13). Rectus femoris

(14). Vastus medialis

(15). Peroneus longus

(16). Tibialis anterior

(17). Extensor digitorum longus

(18). Pectoralis major

(19). Biceps brachii

(20). Brachialis

(21). Pectineus

(22). Adductor longus

(23). Gracilis

(24). Gastrocnemius

(25). Soleous

Major Muscle From The Back

① _____

② _____

③ _____

④ _____

⑤ _____

⑥ _____

⑦ _____

⑧ _____

⑨ _____

Hamstring group

⑩ _____

⑪ _____

⑫ _____

⑬ _____

⑭ _____

⑮ _____

⑯ _____

⑰ _____

⑱ _____

⑲ _____

⑳ _____

Major Muscle From The Back
- Answer -

(1). Occipitalis

(2). Stemocleoidomastoid

(3). Trapezius

(4). Deltoid

(5). Latissimus dorsi

(6). External abdominal oblique

(7). Gluteus medius

(8). Gluteus maximus

(9). Adductor magnus

(10). Semitendinosus

(11). Biceps femoris

(12). Semimembranosus

(13). Achilles tendon

(14). Triceps brachii

(15). Extensor digitorum

(16). Extensor carpi group

(17). Gastrocnemius

(18). Soleus

(19). Peroneus brevis

(20). Peroneus longus

Muscles of Lower Leg

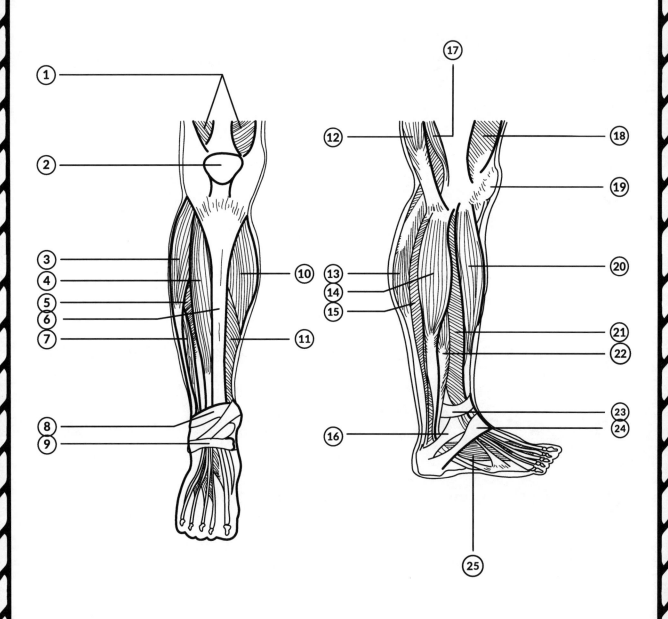

Muscles of Lower Leg
- Answer -

(1). Quadriceps femoris

(2). Patella

(3). Peroneus longus

(4). Tibialis anterior

(5). Extensor digitorum longus

(6). Tibia

(7). Extensor hallucis longus

(8). Superior extensor retinaculum

(9). Inferior extensor retinaculum

(10). Gastrocnemius

(11). Soleus

(12). Biceps femoris

(13). Gastrocnemius

(14). Peroneus longus

(15). Soleus

(16). Superior peroneal retinaculum

(17). Vastus lateralis

(18). Quadriceps femoris

(19). Patella

(20). Tibialis anterior

(21). Extensor digitorum longus

(22). Peroneus brevis

(23). Superior extensor retinaculum

(24). Inferior extensor retinaculum

(25). Extensor digitorum brevis

Muscles of The Posterior Lower Leg

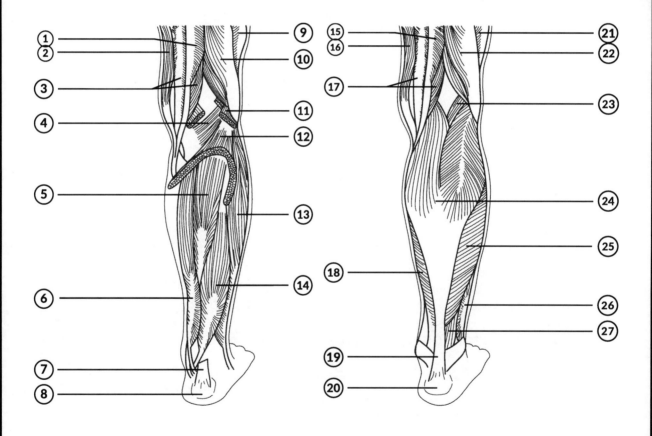

Muscles of The Posterior Lower Leg
- Answer -

(1). Semitendinosus

(2). Graciilis

(3). Semimembranosus

(4). Popliteus

(5). Tibialis posterior

(6). Flexor digitorum longus

(7). Achilles tendon

(8). Calcaneous

(9). Vastus lateralis

(10). Biceps femoris

(11). Gastrocnemius

(12). Soleus

(13). Peroneus longus

(14). Flexor hallucis longus

(15). Semitendinosus

(16). Graciilis

(17). Semimembranosus

(18). Soleus

(19). Achilles tendon

(20). Calcaneous

(21). Vastus lateralis

(22). Biceps femoris

(23). Plantaris

(24). Gastrocnemius

(25). Soleus

(26). Peroneus longus

(27). Peroneus brevis

Muscles of the Leg (Calf) and Foot
(and other important landmarks)

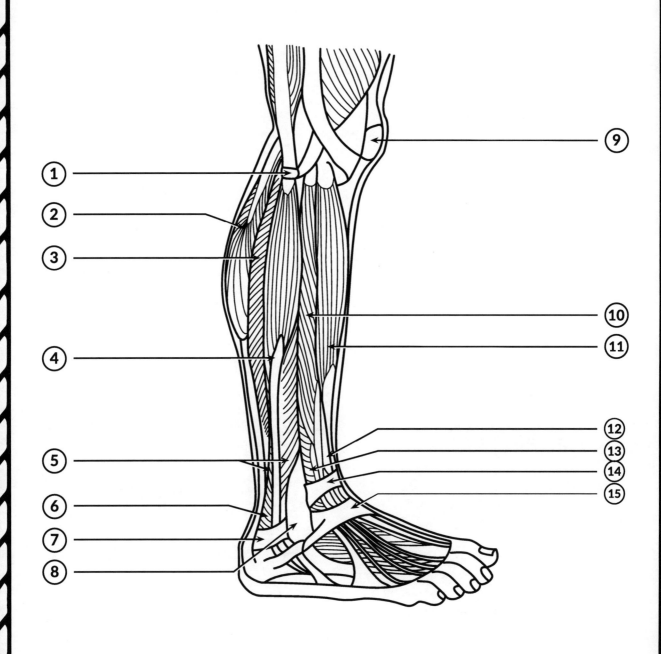

Muscles of the Leg (Calf) and Foot
(and other important landmarks)
- Answer -

(1). Head of the fibula

(2). Gastrocnemius

(3). Soleus

(4). Peroneus longus

(5). Peroneus brevis

(6). Flexor hallicus longus

(7). Peroneal retinaculum

(8). Lateral malleolus ("ankle bone")

(9). Patella

(10). Extensor digitorum longus

(11). Tibialis anterior

(12). Tensor hallicus longus

(13). Peroneus tertius

(14). Superior extensor retinaculum

(15). Inferior extensor retinaculum

Muscles of the Anterior Thigh
(and other important landmarks)

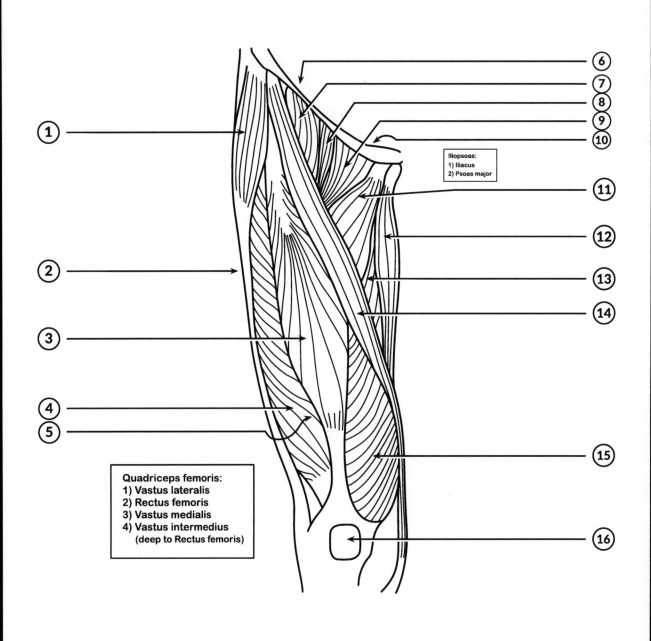

Iliopsoas:
1) Iliacus
2) Psoas major

Quadriceps femoris:
1) Vastus lateralis
2) Rectus femoris
3) Vastus medialis
4) Vastus intermedius
   (deep to Rectus femoris)

Muscles of the Anterior Thigh
(and other important landmarks)
- Answer -

(1). Tensor fasciae lata

(2). (Iliotibial tract)

(3). Rectus femoris

(4). Vastus lateralis

(5). Vastus intermedius
(deep to rectus femoris)

(6). (Inguinal ligament)

(7). Iliacus

(8). Psoas major

(9). Pectineus

(10). Adductor brevis
(deep beneath pectineus)

(11). Adductor longus

(12). Gracilus

(13). Adductor magnus

(14). Sartorius

(15). Vastus medialis

(16). (Patella)

Muscles of the Posterior Thigh
(and other important landmarks)

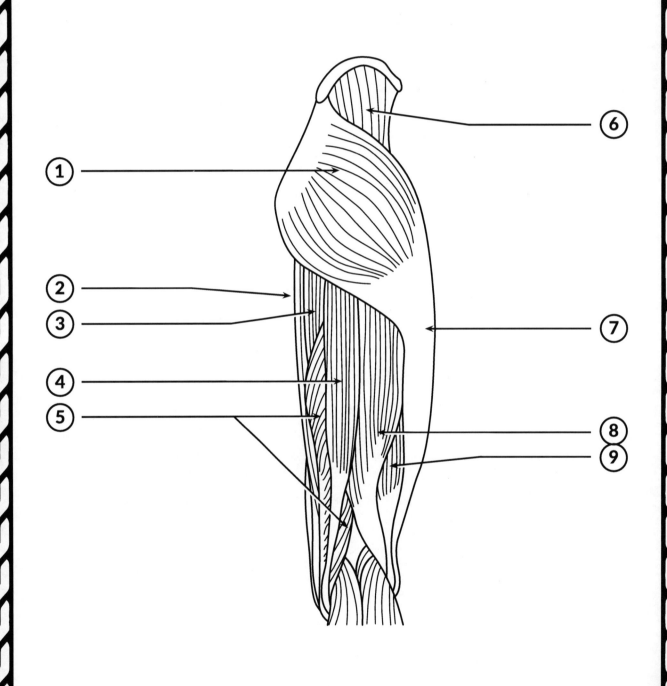

Muscles of the Posterior Thigh
(and other important landmarks)
- Answer -

(1). Gluteus maximus

(2). Gracilis

(3). Adductor magnus

(4). Semitendinosus

(5). Semimembranosus

(6). Gluteus medius

(7). (Iliotibial tract)

(8). Biceps femoris:
Long head

(9). Short head

Muscles of Abdomen

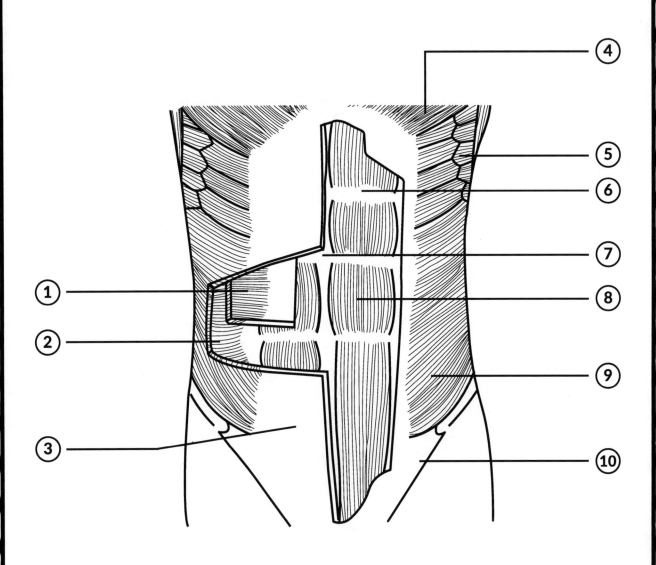

Muscles of Abdomen
- Answer -

(1). Transversus abdominis

(2). Internal oblique

(3). Aponeurosis

(4). Pectoralis major

(5). Serratus anterior

(6). Tendinous intersection

(7). Linea alba

(8). Rectus abdominis

(9). External oblique

(10). Inguinal ligament

Neck and Shoulder Muscles

Anterior

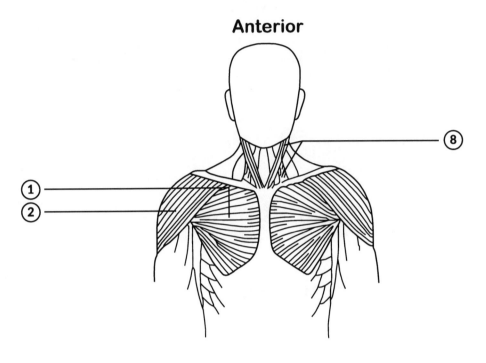

Posterior

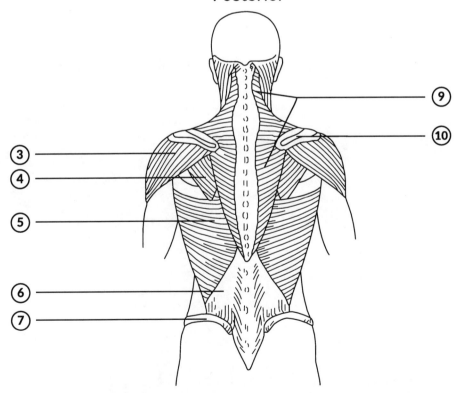

Neck and Shoulder Muscles
- Answer -

(1). Pectoralis major

(2). Deltoid

(3). Deltoid

(4). Infraspinatus

(5). Latissimus dorsi

(6). Lumbar aponeurosis

(7). Iliac crest (of hip bone)

(8). Sternocleidomastoid

(9). Trapezius

(10). Spine of scapula

Name of Muscles

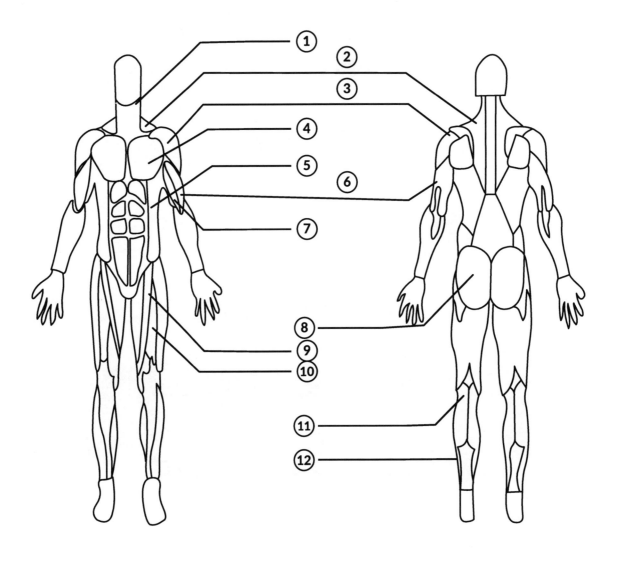

Name of Muscles
- Answer -

(1). Sternocleidomastoid

(2). Trapezius

(3). Deltoid

(4). Pectoralis Major

(5). External Oblique

(6). Triceps brachii

(7). Biceps brachii

(8). Gluteus maximus

(9). Sartorius

(10). Adductor longus

(11). Gastrocnemius

(12). Soleus

Neck and Torso Muscles

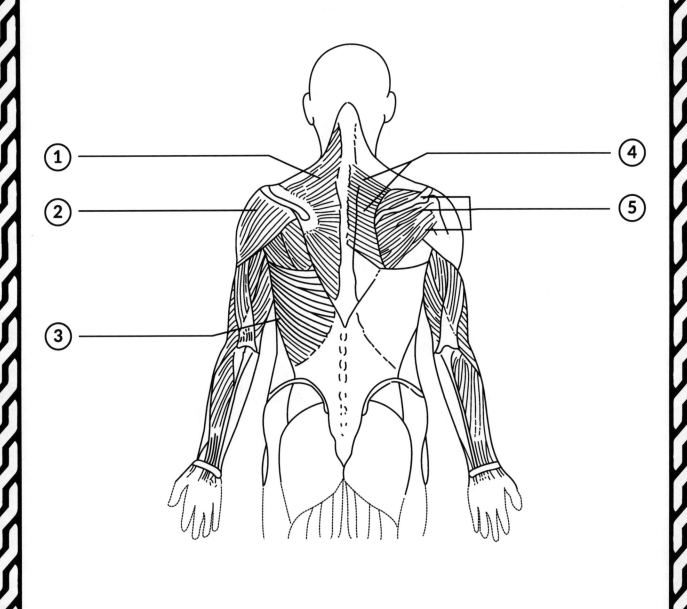

Neck and Torso Muscles

- Answer -

(1). Trapezius

(2). Deltoid

(3). Latissimus dorsi

(4). Rhomboids

(5). Rotator cuff muscles

Muscles of The Neck

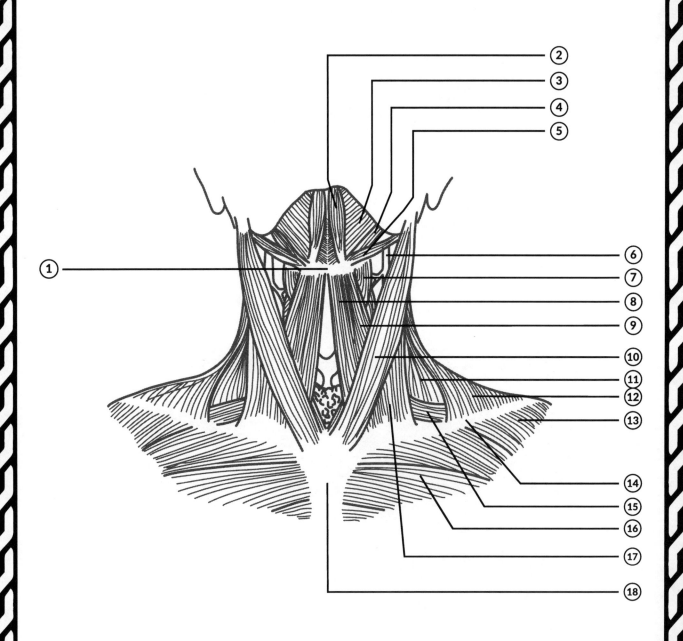

Muscles of The Neck
- Answer -

(1). Hyoid bone

(2). Digastric

(3). Mylohyoid

(4). Stylohyoid

(5). Digastric

(6). Jugular vein

(7). Thyrohyoid

(8). Sternohyoid

(9). Omohyoid

(10). Sternocleidomastoid

(11). Scalenes

(12). Trapezius

(13). Deltoid

(14). Clavicle bone

(15). Omohyoid

(16). Pectoralis major

(17). Sternocleidomastoid

(18). Sternum bone

A Closer Look at Skeletal Muscle Anatomy

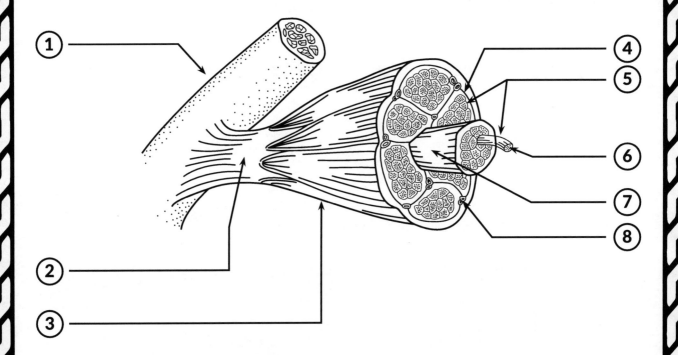

A Closer Look at Skeletal Muscle Anatomy
- Answer -

(1). Bone

(2). Tendon

(3). Epimysium

(4). Perimysium

(5). Endomysium

(6). Muscle fiber

(7). Muscle fascicle

(8). Blood vessel

Back Muscles

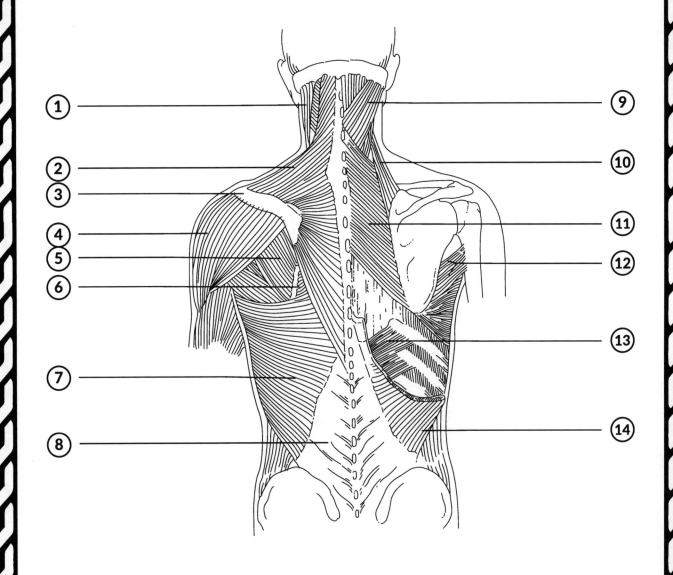

1

2

3

4

5

6

7

8

9

10

11

12

13

14

Back Muscles
- Answer -

(1). Sternocleidomastoid (SCM)

(2). Trapezius

(3). Acromion

(4). Deltoid

(5). Infraspinatus

(6). Rhomboid major

(7). Latissimus dorsi

(8). Thoracolumbar fascia

(9). Splenius capitus

(10). Levator scapulae

(11). Rhomboid major

(12). Teres minor and major

(13). Serratus posterior inferior

(14). Lumbar triangle

Trapezius

Trapezius
- Answer -

(1). Occipital bone

(2). Thoracic vertebra

(3). Trapezius muscle

(4). Scapula

Chest and Abdomen

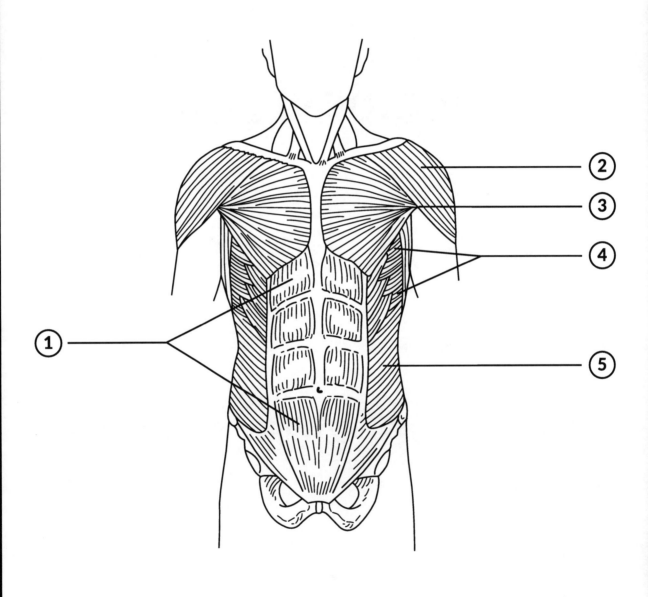

Chest and Abdomen
- Answer -

(1). Rectus abdominis
(covered by rectus sheath)

(2). Deltoid

(3). Pectoralis major

(4). Serratus anterior

(5). External oblique

Anterior Muscles of The Chest and Abdomen

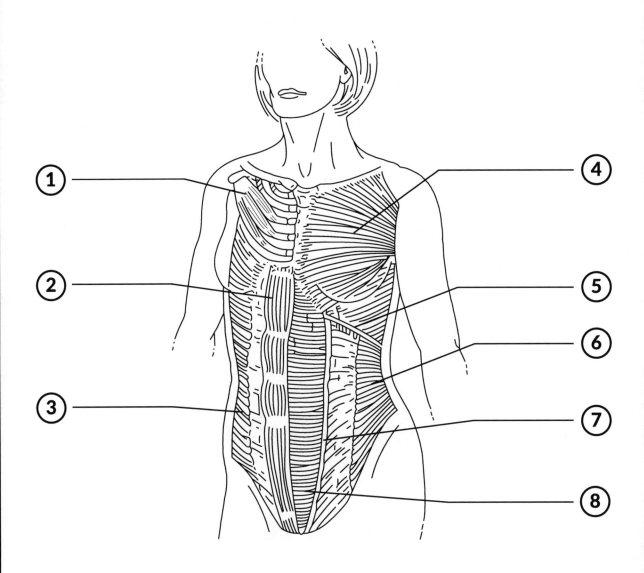

Anterior Muscles of The Chest and Abdomen
- Answer -

(1). Pectoralis minor

(2). Rectus abdominis

(3). External oblique

(4). Pectoralis major

(5). Cut edge of external oblique

(6). Internal oblique

(7). Cut edge of aponeurosis
of internal oblique

(8). Transversus abdominis

Deep Muscles of the Gluteal Region of the Posterior Thigh

(and other important landmarks)

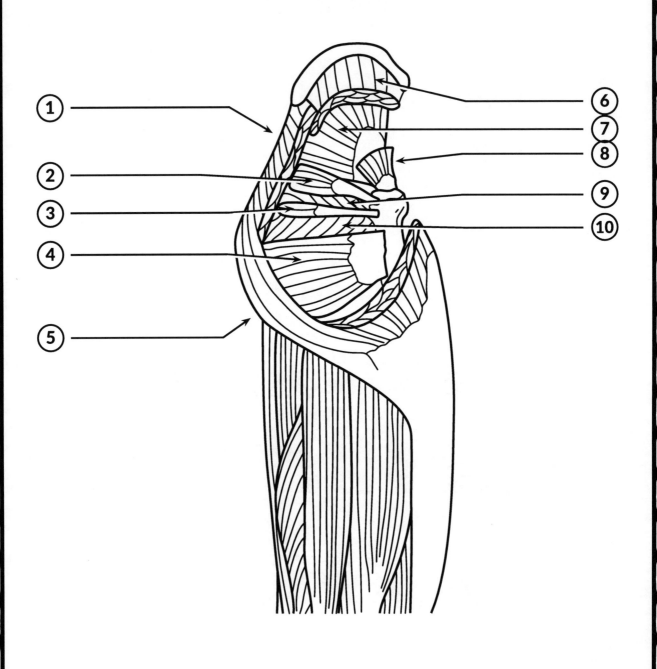

① ② ③ ④ ⑤

⑥ ⑦ ⑧ ⑨ ⑩

Deep Muscles of the Gluteal Region of the Posterior Thigh
(and other important landmarks)

- Answer -

(1). Gluteus maximus

(2). Piriformis

(3). Obturator internus

(4). Obturator externus

(5). Gluteus maximus

(6). Gluteus medius

(7). Gluteus minimus

(8). Gluteus medius

(9). Superior gemellus

(10). Inferior gemellus

Muscles of The Face

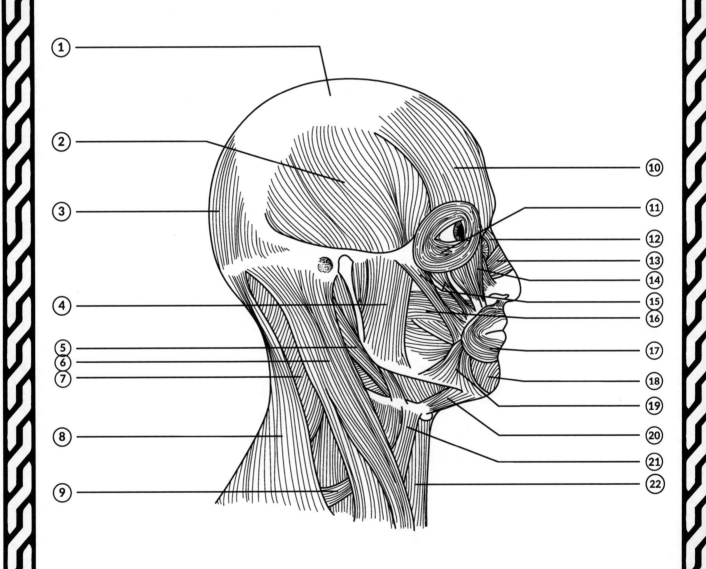

Muscles of The Face
- Answer -

(1). Epicranial aponeurosis

(2). Temporalis

(3). Occipitalis

(4). Masseter

(5). Digastric

(6). Sternocleidomastoid

(7). Spenius capitus

(8). Trapezius

(9). Omohyoid

(10). Frontalis

(11). Orbicularis oculi

(12). Procerus

(13). Nasalis

(14). Levator labii superioris

(15). Zygomaticus

(16). Buccinator

(17). Orbicularis oris

(18). Mentalis

(19). Depressor anguli oris

(20). Digastric

(21). Omohyoid

(22). Sternohyoid

Facial Muscles

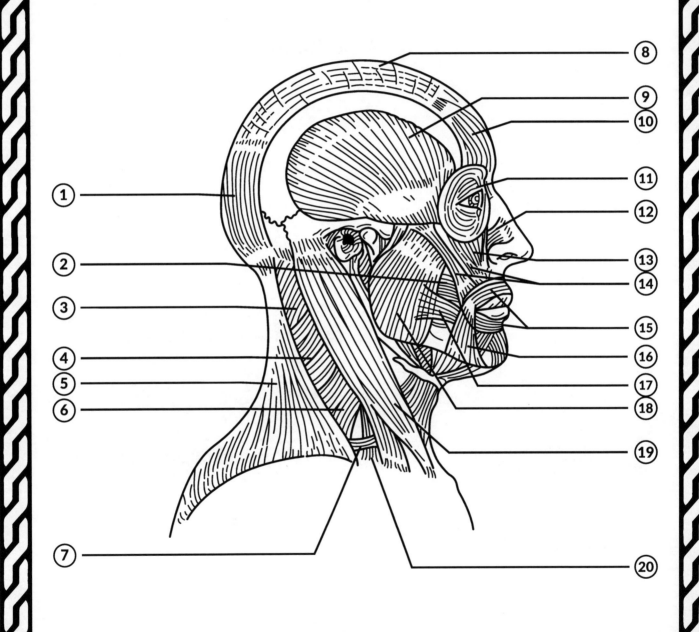

Facial Muscles
- Answer -

(1). Occipitalis

(2). Buccinator

(3). Splenius capitus

(4). Levator scapulae

(5). Trapezius

(6). Middle scalene

(7). Omonyoid

(8). Cranial aponeurosis

(9). Temporalis

(10). Frontalis

(11). Orbicularis oculi

(12). Levator labii superioris alaque nasi

(13). Levator labii superioris

(14). Zygomaticus major and minor

(15). Orbicularis oris

(16). Depressor anguli oris

(17). Risorius

(18). Masseter

(19). Sternocleidomastoid

(20). Anterior scalene

Facial Muscles

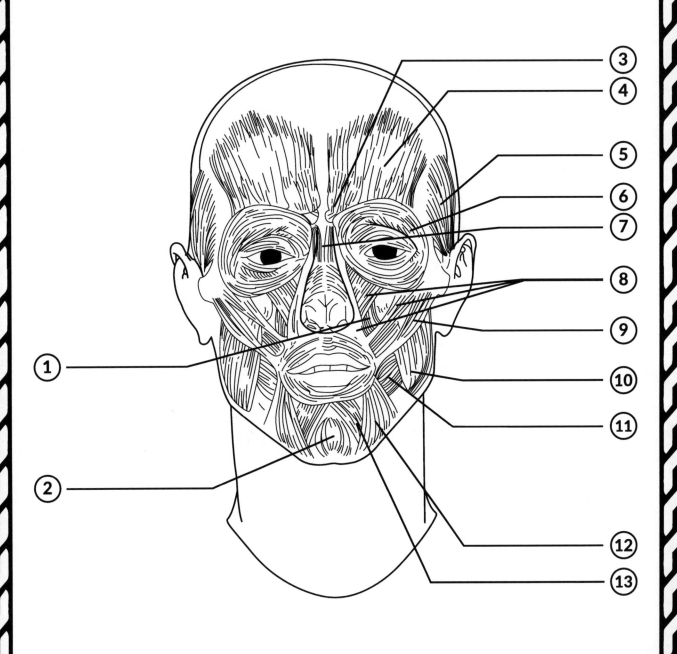

① ② ③ ④ ⑤ ⑥ ⑦ ⑧ ⑨ ⑩ ⑪ ⑫ ⑬

Facial Muscles
- Answer -

(1). Caninus

(2). Mentalis

(3). Corrugator

(4). Frontalis

(5). Temporalis

(6). Orbicularis oculi

(7). Procerus

(8). Quadratus labii superioris

(9). Zygomaticus major

(10). Masseter

(11). Buccinator

(12). Triangularis

(13). Depressor labii inferioris

Facial Muscles

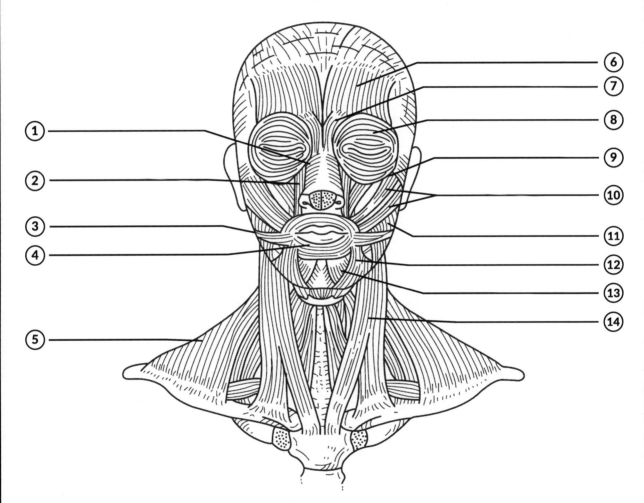

Note: Sternocleidomastoid has two parts.

Facial Muscles
- Answer -

(1). Nasalis

(2). Levator labii superioris alaque nasi

(3). Risorius

(4). Orbicularis oris

(5). Trapezius

(6). Frontalis

(7). Corrugator supercilii

(8). Orbicularis oculi

(9). Levator labii superioris

(10). Zygomaticus major and minor

(11). Masseter

(12). Depressor anguli oris

(13). Mentalis

(14). Sternocleidomastoid

Muscle Types

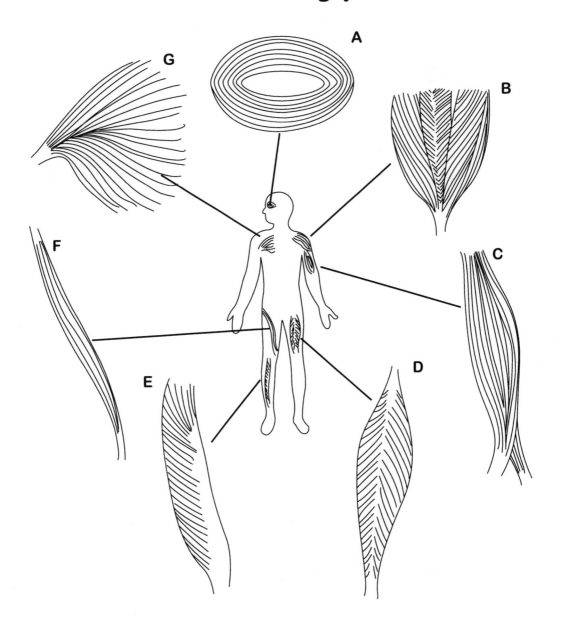

- Answer -

(A). Circular

(B). Multipennate

(C). Fusiform

(D). Bipennate

(E). Unipennate

(F). Parallel

(G). Convergent

Joints

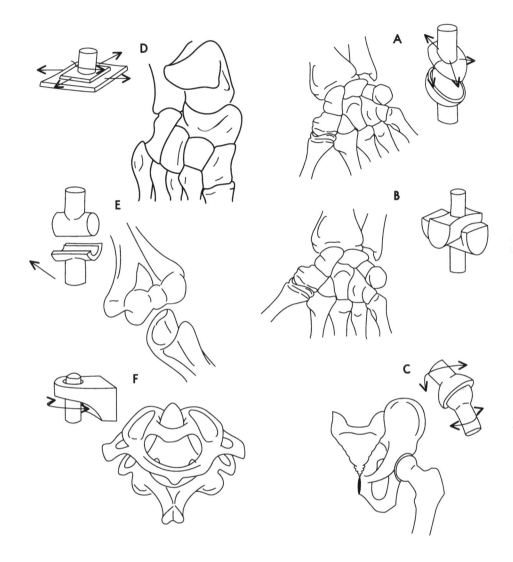

- Answer -

(A). Condyloid joint

(B). Saddle joint

(C). Ball-and-socket joint

(D). Gliding joint

(E). Hinge joint

(F). Pivot joint

Made in the USA
Monee, IL
13 September 2022

13916993R00046